NUTRITION DURING PREGNANCY

Irina Fomina

INTRODUCTION:

Nourishing Your Journey Through Pregnancy

In general, eating "real food" is considered a healthy activity. However, the notion of genuine food is a fuzzy area within nutrition. Here are a few methods to judge how "real" your diet is.

Nutrient-rich foods, sometimes referred to as nutrient-dense foods, contain numerous nutrients. Nutrients are split into two categories: Macronutrients, which comprise carbs, proteins, and fats, and micronutrients, which include vitamins and minerals If a food is high in vitamins, minerals, fiber, protein, and/or beneficial fatty acids, it is deemed nutrient-rich. On the flip side, if the meal does not include many of these components, it is termed nutrient-poor. Most genuine foods are nutrient-dense foods that help fuel your body.

Whole foods are foods that are ingested similarly to how they appear in nature. Most entire foods do not contain added sugars, processed carbs, added colors or tastes, or other synthetic additives. Most entire foods are inherently nutrient-dense; genuine foods include fruits, vegetables, nuts, seeds, legumes, dairy, meat, poultry, and seafood.

Unprocessed foods, like whole foods, are not manipulated, and they seem identical to how they do in nature. In current civilization, many meals are processed until they are scarcely identifiable from their original form and wouldn't satisfy the actual food criteria.

- ### The Importance of Nutrition During Pregnancy

Congratulations on commencing this beautiful adventure of pregnancy! The following nine months will be full of joy, difficulties, and numerous moments of suspense. One of the most crucial components of this trip is ensuring that you supply your body and your baby with the finest possible nourishment. Welcome to "Nourishing Your Journey Through Pregnancy," a complete guide to understanding and embracing the power of nutrition during this transforming period.

- ### How This Book Can Help You

Pregnancy is a season of tremendous change and growth both for you and the life you are nourishing. As your body goes through extraordinary modifications to accommodate the new life within, it requires an additional dosage of care and food. Proper nutrition is the cornerstone of a healthy pregnancy, delivering advantages that extend long beyond these nine months.

In this book, we'll dig into the important nutrients your body needs to promote the development of your baby's brain, bones, and overall well-being. We'll discuss the ins and outs of meal planning, tackling typical difficulties like morning sickness and food cravings, and adapting to the changing requirements of your body.

But this book isn't simply about charts and lists. It's about equipping you with knowledge so that you can make educated decisions regarding your food and health. We'll explore the necessity of hydration, regulating weight gain, and the value of exercise in keeping a healthy and vibrant pregnancy.

Whether you're a first-time parent or well-experienced on the road to motherhood, this book is here to encourage you every step of the way. From learning the importance of folic acid to establishing nutrient-rich meal plans and discovering tasty recipes, "Nourishing Your Journey Through Pregnancy" is your trusty companion on this remarkable experience.

Remember, every pregnancy is unique, and this book is meant to offer you the skills and insights to personalize your nutrition path to your requirements. Let's go on this journey together and guarantee that you and your kid flourish in the most nutritious way possible.

In the following chapters, we'll discuss the vital nutrients, meal planning tactics, unique concerns, and practical recommendations to make your pregnancy a period of optimal well-being. Here's to a healthy and enjoyable pregnant adventure!

CHAPTER ONE

Understanding Pregnancy Nutrition

- ### Nutritional Needs and Changes During Pregnancy

From the moment you find you're expecting, your body starts a spectacular time of development and metamorphosis. Understanding the dietary demands and changes that accompany pregnancy is vital for both your well-being and the growth of your baby.

The Miracle of Pregnancy: Nurturing Two Lives

Pregnancy is an awe-inspiring experience when your body becomes a shelter for new life. It's a period of tremendous change, and your body responds with modifications that support the growth and development of your kid. The increase in blood volume assures an adequate supply of oxygen and nutrients to both you and your baby. Your metabolism changes to supply the energy necessary for the various phases of pregnancy, from the early days of cell division to the latter months of fetal development.

Caloric and Energy Requirements

As your baby develops, so do your caloric and energy demands. It's crucial to find a balance between satisfying your appetite and ensuring that your kid obtains the nutrients necessary for healthy growth. Your body's energy expenditure increases, notably throughout the second and third trimesters. This implies you may need to consume additional calories to fulfill these needs.

However, it's not a license to indulge in bad meals. The quality of calories counts just as much as the number. Opt for nutrient-dense foods that supply the vitamins, minerals, and macronutrients your body demands. A well-rounded diet that includes a mix of fruits, vegetables, whole grains, lean meats, and healthy fats can help you satisfy your nutritional needs.

- ### Key Nutrients for a Healthy Pregnancy

Certain nutrients play major roles throughout pregnancy, and they contribute considerably to the development of your baby's organs, brain, and overall health. Ensuring that you're consuming these nutrients at suitable levels is vital for a successful pregnant journey.

Folic Acid: The Foundation of Early Development

Folic acid, a B vitamin, is a cornerstone of early pregnancy nutrition. It's well-known for its function in avoiding neural tube abnormalities, which disrupt the development of the baby's spinal cord and brain. Adequate folic acid consumption before conception and during the early weeks of pregnancy is necessary. Leafy greens, fortified cereals, citrus fruits, and legumes are great sources of folic acid.

Iron: Ensuring Oxygen Supply and Healthy Growth

Iron takes center stage during pregnancy due to its crucial function in making red blood cells, which deliver oxygen to both you and your growing baby. As your blood volume grows, your iron demands rise as well. Iron deficiency can develop into anemia, making you weary and compromising the transport of oxygen to your baby. Lean meats, chicken, fish, beans, and fortified grains are great sources of iron.

Calcium: Building Strong Bones and Teeth

Calcium is vital for your baby's bone and teeth growth, and it's also important for preserving your bone health. Your baby will drain calcium from your bones if your intake is inadequate, potentially harming your bone density. Dairy products, leafy greens, fortified plant-based milk, and calcium-enriched meals are fantastic providers of this crucial mineral.

Omega-3 Fatty Acids: Nourishing Brain and Vision

Omega-3 fatty acids, particularly DHA (docosahexaenoic acid), are critical for your baby's brain and visual development. These healthy fats also boost your cardiovascular health and may even reduce certain pregnancy-related discomforts. Fatty fish like salmon and trout, walnuts, flaxseeds, and chia seeds are great sources of omega-3 fatty acids.

Understanding the nuances of pregnancy nutrition allows you to make educated decisions that positively influence both you and your baby. By identifying the changes your body takes and the necessary nutrients it requires, you're well on your way to laying a foundation of health for this magnificent adventure.

CHAPTER TWO

Building a Balanced Diet: Nourishing Your Pregnancy

Congratulations on taking the proactive step of realizing the significance of a balanced diet during pregnancy. As you traverse the extraordinary adventure of fostering new life, ensuring that your body obtains the correct nutrients in the right amounts is crucial. In this part, we will dig into the fundamental concepts of a healthy pregnancy diet, studying the foundations of meal planning and the necessity of portion management.

- **The Basics of a Balanced Pregnancy Diet**

Maintaining a balanced diet is a cornerstone of improving your well-being and the health of your growing kid. A balanced pregnancy diet delivers the vital nutrients required for healthy fetal growth, supports your energy demands, and aids in managing any pregnancy discomforts. Here's a summary of the major components of a healthy pregnancy diet:

Variety of Nutrient-Rich Foods
Diverse dietary choices guarantee that you acquire a variety of vitamins, minerals, and nutrients. Include a wide array of fruits and vegetables, whole grains, lean meats, and healthy fats in your diet. Each food category has specific advantages, contributing to the complete nourishment of both you and your baby.

Adequate Protein Intake
Protein plays a key part in the creation of cells, tissues, and organs. During pregnancy, your protein demands rise to support the development of your baby's organs, muscles, and placenta. Lean meats, poultry, fish, eggs, lentils, and dairy products are great sources of protein.

Complex Carbohydrates
Complex carbs, found in whole grains, fruits, and vegetables, give a consistent supply of energy. They also include fiber, which assists with digestion and avoids constipation—a typical problem during pregnancy.

Healthy Fats
Healthy fats are necessary for your baby's brain and nervous system development. Incorporate sources of omega-3 fatty acids, such as fatty fish, walnuts, flaxseeds, and chia seeds, into your diet. Avocados, almonds, and olive oil are other fantastic sources of healthy fats.

Calcium-Rich Foods
Calcium is vital for your baby's bone growth and sustaining your bone health. Dairy products, fortified plant-based milk, leafy greens, and calcium-enriched meals guarantee you satisfy your calcium needs.

Iron-Rich Choices
As described in the preceding section, iron is important for oxygen transport. Incorporate iron-rich foods including lean meats, chicken, fish, lentils, and fortified cereals to prevent iron deficiency and anemia.

Hydration
Staying hydrated is vital for maintaining amniotic fluid levels and sustaining your body's increasing blood volume. Aim to drink lots of water throughout the day and consider including hydrating items like fruits and vegetables in your meals.

- ## Meal Planning and Portion Control

Efficient meal planning and portion management are crucial measures for keeping a balanced and healthy pregnant diet. These techniques allow you to give your body the nutrition it needs while regulating weight growth healthily.

1. Designing Nutrient-Rich Meals

Crafting meals that are nutrient-rich and well-balanced is the basis of a good pregnant diet. Begin by constructing a meal template that contains a range of items from different dietary categories. Incorporate a source of protein, such as lean meats, poultry, fish, beans, or tofu, to promote the growth of your baby's cells and tissues.

Complex carbs from whole grains, fruits, and vegetables deliver sustained energy and key elements like fiber and vitamins. Don't shy away from healthy fats like avocados, almonds, and olive oil, which help your baby's brain development and general wellness.

Vegetables and fruits should form a considerable portion of each meal. Their rich hues are indicative of the vast spectrum of vitamins and minerals they supply. Aim to fill half your plate with these bright selections

2. Frequent, Smaller Meals

Pregnancy frequently comes with alterations in appetite and digestion. To negotiate these shifts, consider eating smaller, more frequent meals throughout the day. This strategy not only helps control discomforts like morning sickness and heartburn but also delivers a consistent supply of nutrition to you and your baby.

By spreading out your meals, you may maintain more stable energy levels, minimizing severe hunger that can contribute to overeating. Opt for balanced snacks like Greek yogurt with berries, a handful of almonds and dried fruits, or whole-grain crackers with hummus.

3. **Snacking Smartly**

Smart snacking between meals can play a key part in your pregnancy diet. Snacks help bridge the gap between meals and give a chance to include additional nutrients. When picking snacks, go for foods that include a combination of protein, healthy fats, and complex carbs.

Fruits are a fantastic choice, giving natural sweetness and a variety of micronutrients. Pairing fruits with a source of protein, such as a tiny piece of cheese or a handful of nuts, may make for a pleasant and healthy snack.

4. Mindful Portion Control

While pregnancy is not a time for severe calorie tracking or restrictive eating, being careful of portion sizes can help you manage your nutritional intake. Tune attention to your body's cues of hunger and fullness. Eat till you're pleasantly content rather than too stuffed.

Use visual clues to direct your portions. For example, a meal of protein should be around the size of your palm, while a serving of carbs should be roughly the size of your fist. Including a variety of foods in proper quantities ensures you're getting the optimal combination of nutrients.

5. Planning for Cravings

Cravings during pregnancy are a reality for many pregnant moms. While it's alright to indulge occasionally, try finding healthier options for your desires. If you're looking for something sweet, opt for a piece of fruit; if you're seeking something savory, consider whole-grain crackers with hummus.

Remember, giving in to desires periodically is entirely natural and may be a source of delight. The key is moderation and ensuring that your entire diet remains balanced and nourishing.

6. Seeking Professional Guidance

As you commence on this path of developing a healthy pregnancy diet, it's vital to know that individual needs might differ. If you're concerned about your food choices or have specific concerns, consider visiting a registered dietitian or healthcare practitioner who specializes in prenatal nutrition. They can give specialized assistance targeted to your specific situation.

By adopting meal planning and portion management, you're taking proactive efforts to supply your body and baby with the nutrition they require. These practices create a firm basis for a healthy, pleasurable, and rewarding pregnant experience.

CHAPTER THREE

Essential Nutrients for Pregnancy: Nurturing Life's Foundation

As you start on this magnificent adventure of pregnancy, understanding the vital nutrients that play a critical part in your baby's growth and well-being becomes a light of information guiding you forward. This section provides a detailed analysis of four critical nutrients that deserve not just attention, but a place of importance, during this changing moment.

• Folic Acid and Folate-Rich Foods: Building Blocks of Development

Folic acid, a B vitamin known for its relevance, ranks as one of the most critical nutrients throughout pregnancy. Its significance in the early phases of development, particularly when the neural tube forms—later becoming the spinal cord and brain—is important.

The pursuit of appropriate folic acid consumption should ideally start before pregnancy. The suggested technique is introducing folate-rich foods into your diet. These include an assortment of nature's treasures—leafy green vegetables like spinach and kale, brilliant citrus fruits alive with energy, legumes loaded with sustenance, and grains fortified to boost your journey into motherhood.

Understanding folic acid's involvement in preventing neural tube abnormalities highlights its relevance. The neural tube forms within the first month of pregnancy, frequently before you even realize you're pregnant. By adopting folate-rich meals, you're laying the groundwork for a robust foundation of growth.

• Iron-Rich Foods for Preventing Anemia: Oxygenation for Two

Within the symphony of pregnancy's complex changes, iron takes center stage. Its crucial significance in regulating hemoglobin levels—the very protein within red blood cells that orchestrates the delivery of oxygen throughout your body—is apparent.

The requirement for iron climbs as your blood volume increases considerably during pregnancy. Neglecting this need can lead to iron deficiency anemia, a condition characterized by signs of weariness, weakness, and increased susceptibility to infections.

To resist this, embrace the inclusion of iron-rich meals. Delight in the breadth of alternatives available—lean meats and poultry, a marine dance of fish, the substantial sustenance of beans and lentils, and even fortified cereals that are champions of this crucial mineral. To improve iron absorption, examine the symphony of vitamin C-rich meals that elegantly enhance its intake.

As you pay attention to the significance of iron in oxygenation, visualize the cascade of energy it bestows onto both you and your developing kid. From the orchestration of cellular activities to the maintenance of a robust immune system, iron's contribution is a ringing song of life.

• Calcium and Bone Health: Strong Foundations for Both

As the orchestrator of bone and tooth growth for your infant, calcium stands as an architectural cornerstone. But its importance extends beyond your baby's demands; your bone health intertwines with the calcium tale.

In the delicate tapestry of pregnancy, if your diet lacks sufficient calcium, your body, in its amazing wisdom, will draw into your bone reserves to satisfy your baby's demands. This interchange, however a monument to the body's resiliency, highlights the significance of keeping your bone density.

Traditional sources of calcium, such as the offers of dairy—milk, yogurt, cheese—stand steadfast. For individuals who tread a plant-based road, the domain of fortified plant-based milk, leafy greens overflowing in vitality, and the mosaic of almonds and chia seeds bring peace. A ballet of calcium-rich alternatives awaits, nourishing both you and your baby's growth.

• Omega-3 Fatty Acids for Brain Development: Nourishing the Mind

Within the domain of nutrition, omega-3 fatty acids hold a symphony of advantages, with docosahexaenoic acid (DHA) taking center stage. Its profound influence on brain and eyesight development for your infant is awe-inspiring.

DHA, a master of cell membrane composition in the brain and eyes, is a driving factor behind their growth and operation. The marine realm offers us the richness of fatty fish—salmon, mackerel, and trout—as unequaled sources of DHA. Yet, the plant kingdom offers its treasures, encased in the shapes of walnuts, flaxseeds, and chia seeds.

Embracing these plant-based sources not only nurtures your baby's brain development but also increases your well-being. Omega-3 fatty acids have been associated with lower inflammation, perhaps easing some of the discomforts that often accompany pregnancy.

Incorporating these critical nutrients into your prenatal diet guarantees that you're giving your baby a firm foundation for growth and development while also supporting your health. As you pick and prepare foods, bear in mind that each nutrient has a particular purpose, adding to the extraordinary adventure you're doing.

CHAPTER FOUR

Protein and Energy Needs: Fueling Life's Creation

Amidst the awe and wonder of pregnancy, the subtle dance of sustenance becomes vital. This part goes deep into the dynamic interaction of protein and energy, two pillars that drive the path of fostering life within.

- ### Protein-Rich Foods for Growth and Development

In the vast symphony of creation, protein takes on a function analogous to that of a master composer. It orchestrates the delicate melodies of growth and development, sculpting the very essence of your baby's existence. During pregnancy, protein-rich meals climb to a place of prominence, becoming the building blocks that form the basis for your baby's extraordinary adventure.

Imagine the miracle of lean meats—chicken, turkey, and other poultry—each mouthful filled with high-quality protein. These meats, replete with important amino acids, help the creation of your baby's cells and tissues. The blend of tastes and nutrients they give encourages you to embark on a gourmet voyage of nurturing sustenance.

Fish, a seafaring treasure trove, lends its wealth to your pregnant plate. The omega-3 fatty acids in salmon and the protein-packed nutrition of tuna reward your body and baby with a symphony of nutrients. However, a word of caution: Choose fish that are low in mercury to ensure both your well-being and your baby's growth.

Eggs, a versatile nutritional marvel, extend their embrace to both protein and choline—an vital ingredient that promotes the delicate tapestry of brain development. Dairy products, equally rich in protein and calcium, become the epitome of dual feeding, supporting bone health and growth.

Venturing into the luxuriant expanse of plant life, beans and lentils take center stage. These legumes, analogous to nature's pearls, constitute a symphony of protein, fiber, and folate—a composition that vibrates with sustenance, energy, and caring.

- ### Managing Energy Intake and Weight Gain

Within the delicate mosaic of pregnancy, the energy you pump into your body becomes the brushstroke that paints the canvas of your journey. The demands alter and fluctuate as you transit the trimesters, each one signifying a particular crescendo of your body's growth.

The second and third trimesters frequently herald a rise in energy requirements, reflecting the amazing symphony of growth and development. However, this increase is not an invitation to indulge indiscriminately, but rather a chance to embrace the ideals of mindful nutrition.

Imagine your diet as a palette, each meal expressing a hue of nourishment. Fruits and vegetables give brilliant colors of vitamins and minerals, while lean proteins contribute depth and structure. Whole grains weave intricacy into the composition, and healthy fats lend a touch of richness.

Navigating this creative masterpiece entails a precise tango between energy expenditure and intake. Engaging in targeted physical exercise, aligned with your specific requirements and skills, harmonizes these factors. By tuning into your body's signs, you're able to build a symphony of balanced energy use.

Weight gain, a visible manifestation of your path, emerges at the forefront. While it's an intrinsic aspect of pregnancy, controlling it becomes a creative endeavor. Swift weight gain can bring the danger of difficulties, highlighting the significance of a controlled approach.

As you navigate this environment, let the rhythms of your body lead you. Recognize the whispers of hunger and the indications of satiety. Make choices that favor nutrient density and satiety, embracing nourishment that resonates with both your well-being and the blossoming life inside you.

Protein and energy—are two dynamic forces that blend with the song of pregnancy. By embracing the orchestra of protein-rich meals and balancing energy intake, you're not only fuelling physical growth; you're fostering the very essence of vigor and life.

CHAPTER FIVE

Hydration and Fluid Intake: Nourishing Life's Flow

Within the tapestry of pregnancy, the essence of hydration and fluid intake emerges as a river of energy. This part immerses us in the necessity of remaining hydrated during this transforming journey and goes into the art of selecting healthy fluid alternatives.

• Importance of Staying Hydrated During Pregnancy

Imagine water as the vital lifeblood that feeds you and your growing kid. Staying hydrated takes on a heightened relevance throughout pregnancy as your body navigates a symphony of changes. Fluids perform a diverse role, from promoting the increase of your blood volume to cushioning your baby inside the amniotic fluid.

Dehydration can show in several ways, from increased weariness to dizziness and even consequences like urinary tract infections. Your body, with its sophisticated intelligence, sends subtle signs of thirst that should not be ignored. Paying awareness to these indications provides the cornerstone of a nutritious pregnant journey.

As you travel through the trimesters, your fluid demands alter. The second and third trimesters frequently bring an increased requirement for hydration due to larger blood volume and the amniotic fluid around your baby. Tailoring your fluid intake to your particular demands promotes a smooth flow of nutrients to both you and your baby.

The symphony of hydration echoes beyond your bodily well-being. Proper hydration helps ease typical pregnant discomforts, such as constipation and edema. It also assists in the control of body temperature, a task that becomes more crucial when hormonal changes impact your internal climate.

• Choosing Healthy Fluid Options

Fluid intake surpasses simply hydration; it becomes a route for sustenance. While water gets the major limelight, other healthy fluid alternatives offer a symphony of advantages.

Consider the elegance of herbal teas, giving warmth and comfort amid an assortment of tastes. Opt for caffeine-free choices, as excessive caffeine intake should be controlled during pregnancy. Teas laced with ginger and chamomile can be relaxing companions, reducing pregnant discomforts.

Fruits give their own watery offerings—cucumber, watermelon, and citrus fruits, to mention a few. These fruits are not only hydrating but also rich in vitamins and minerals that enhance your well-being.

Soups, both transparent and broth-based, provide the nutrients of fluids and the comfort of warmth. The technique of producing nutrient-rich broths delivers both hydration and a flavor of gourmet delight.

Coconut water, a natural electrolyte-rich elixir, extends its hand to relieve your thirst. Its delicate flavor, suggestive of tropical retreats, is a tribute to the vast palette of fluid possibilities accessible.

Embrace the flexibility of your choices, knowing that each drink nourishes not just your body but also the life inside. Let your instincts guide you as you make options consistent with your tastes and needs.

By realizing the necessity of being hydrated and cultivating a symphony of healthy fluid alternatives, you're fostering the very essence of life within you. This chapter of your pregnancy experience speaks to the flow of energy, the whispers of well-being, and the flowing beauty of sustenance.

As the journey unfolds, may the symphony of hydration weave a thread of vitality through the canvas of your pregnancy. Your body, a vessel of life, is sustained not just by the nutrition you choose but also by the fluid energy you accept.

CHAPTER SIX

Managing Nausea and Food Aversions: Navigating the Waves

Amidst the lovely journey of pregnancy, the unexpected visitors of sickness and dietary aversions frequently make their presence known. This section navigates the complicated seas of coping with morning sickness and establishing nutritional methods to overcome these aversions.

- **Coping with Morning Sickness**

Morning sickness, however sometimes misnamed due to its proclivity to occur at any hour, is a familiar friend for many pregnant moms. As your body adjusts to the surge of hormones, the waves of nausea and vomiting might become part of your daily routine.

While morning sickness can be unpleasant, it's essential to remember that it's frequently a symptom of a good pregnancy. Despite its frequency, each woman's experience is unique. Some may glide through pregnancy with little to no pain, while others may find themselves experiencing recurrent waves of queasiness.

In this chapter, we cover several ways to help you manage morning sickness. From snacking on small, frequent meals to trying ginger and mint—natural medicines recognized for their relaxing properties—each choice provides a potential lifeboat amidst the stormy waves.

The assistance of your healthcare practitioner is crucial during this time. They may give insights targeted to your unique situation, helping you develop ways that suit your needs. It's also important to remember that although treating morning sickness is key, it's as vital to ensure you're consuming appropriate nutrients. This takes us to the field of dietary methods for managing food aversions.

- **Nutritional Strategies for Overcoming Aversions**

Pregnancy typically ushers in a dance of food aversions—a phenomenon where items formerly adored may suddenly cause a visceral repulsion. This exquisite interplay of taste and fragrance is a tribute to the enormous changes your body is undergoing.

Navigating food aversions entails a fine balance between recognizing your body's instincts and ensuring you acquire the nutrition both you and your baby need. While it's tempting to avoid foods that provoke aversions, it's equally crucial to find inventive methods to get the necessary nutrients into your diet.

Consider the art of meal pairing—blending foods you can tolerate with those that give critical nutrients. If the notion of particular meals produces waves of agony, investigating other preparation methods or simply attempting various textures could give a remedy.

Embracing a range of flavors and sensations may also generate a symphony of possibilities. If the once-beloved salad elicits an aversion, perhaps a flavorful soup or a healthy smoothie can give a more appealing way to sustenance.

Exploring the realm of prenatal vitamins might be another method. While acquiring nutrition through whole meals is preferable, prenatal vitamins can give a safety net, ensuring you're not missing out on critical vitamins and minerals, especially during periods when food aversions are at their greatest.

The path of handling aversions is a reminder of the wonderful subtleties of pregnancy. As you traverse these new seas, bear in mind that flexibility and adaptation are your allies. The idea is to establish a balance that acknowledges your well-being and promotes the growth of your baby.

By understanding the intricacies of morning sickness and the ebb and flow of food aversions, you're embracing the complex nature of pregnancy. This chapter of your journey asks you to listen to your body's messages, experiment with nutritious solutions, and adjust to the symphony of change.

CHAPTER SEVEN

Dealing with Cravings and Healthy Snacking: Nurturing Temptations

In the rich tapestry of pregnancy, appetites develop as amusing companions, bringing you down unexpected roads of desire. This section digs into the subject of understanding pregnant cravings and gives insights into choosing good eating choices.

• Understanding Pregnancy Cravings

Cravings, frequently quirky and surprising, take center stage throughout pregnancy, taking you on a gastronomic adventure that dances between pleasure and nutrition. The appeal of some meals may tug at your senses with a power that transcends comprehension. While these desires might be enticing, they also look into the delicate symphony of your body's requirements.

Pregnancy desires are not only arbitrary whims; they frequently contain hidden signals. The yearning for specific tastes could suggest a lack of certain nutrients. For instance, a longing for citrus can suggest a requirement for vitamin C, while a yearning for red meat could signal a demand for greater iron.

Cravings can also be impacted by hormonal changes, emotional variables, and cultural influences. Acknowledging these dynamics helps you to connect with your urges from a point of inquiry and awareness.

While indulging in desires may be an enjoyable part of your journey, it's crucial to maintain a balance. Moderation and choosing choices that coincide with your overall dietary objectives guarantee that both your appetites and your health are acknowledged.

• Making Smart Snacking Choices

Snacking takes on a new dimension during pregnancy, moving from plain sustenance to an elegant mix of food and enjoyment. This chapter encourages you to explore the realm of smart eating, developing options that quench your appetites while nourishing your well-being.

Begin by embracing the diversity of whole foods. Fruits, a palate of natural sweetness, offer a symphony of vitamins and fiber. Berries, cherries, and sliced melon form the brushstrokes of your snacking canvas, imbuing your body with both taste and vigor.

Nuts and seeds, nature's pocket-sized powerhouses, offer a delicious crunch while supplying healthful fats and protein. However, portion management becomes an art in itself, ensuring you experience its advantages without overindulgence.

Yogurt, a creamy treat, delivers bacteria that support gut health—a critical part of general well-being. Paired with a drizzle of honey and a sprinkle of almonds, it changes into a snack that embraces both sustenance and pleasure.

Vegetables, colorful and fresh, give countless alternatives for imaginative eating. Carrot sticks, bell pepper strips, and cucumber rounds become conduits of water and nutrients. Paired with hummus or a yogurt-based dip, they raise your snacking experience to a symphony of flavors.

Smart eating entails tuning into your body's signs and knowing the distinction between actual hunger and emotional responses. Keeping a range of healthful snacks readily available will empower you to make thoughtful choices when cravings occur.

By interacting with your appetites and navigating the domain of sensible eating, you're participating in the complicated ballet of pregnant nutrition. This stage of your journey allows you to embrace your wants while nurturing your body—a delicate balance that honors both indulgence and wellness.

CHAPTER EIGHT

Special Dietary Considerations: Nurturing Through Choices

In the complicated symphony of pregnancy nutrition, particular dietary factors produce individual melodies that accord with the unique demands of pregnant moms. This section looks into the factors surrounding vegetarian and vegan diets during pregnancy, as well as the necessity of food safety and avoiding dangerous ingredients.

- ## Vegetarian and Vegan Diets During Pregnancy

Vegetarian and vegan diets, rich in plant-based goodness, are chosen for a range of reasons, from ethics to health. However, during pregnancy, these nutritional approaches demand careful attention to assure the feeding of both you and your growing kid.

Vegetarian diets, which eliminate meat but include plant-based foods such as fruits, vegetables, healthy grains, legumes, and dairy, can supply a diversity of nutrients when well-balanced. Protein foods such as beans and dairy can play a crucial role in ensuring healthy growth.

Vegan diets, which ban all animal products, necessitate even more careful attention. While they can be nutritionally sufficient, care is required to guarantee proper consumption of nutrients such as protein, iron, calcium, vitamin B12, omega-3 fatty acids, and zinc. Supplements or fortified meals could become partners in bridging such gaps.

Consulting a healthcare physician or certified dietitian who specializes in prenatal nutrition is crucial while following vegetarian or vegan diets throughout pregnancy. Their counsel can help you develop a strategy that corresponds with your nutritional choices while ensuring your well-being and that of your kid.

- ## Food Safety and Avoiding Harmful Substances

Pregnancy compounds the necessity of food safety since your body's sensitivity to specific microorganisms and toxins rises. This chapter underscores the value of making educated decisions to preserve your health and the well-being of your infant.

Avoiding hazardous drugs extends beyond your eating choices. It involves keeping clear of alcohol, cigarettes, and recreational drugs. These chemicals can have a tremendous influence on your baby's growth and general health.

Additionally, knowing the basics of food safety becomes vital. Unpasteurized dairy products and some raw or undercooked meals raise the risk of foodborne infections, which can have serious implications during pregnancy. Proper food handling, storage, and cleanliness standards are the pillars of protection against these threats.

Fish-eating, while a rich source of omega-3 fatty acids, takes judgment. Certain species of fish can be rich in mercury, a chemical that might disrupt your baby's growing neurological system. Opt for low-mercury fish alternatives and consider including plant-based omega-3 sources such as flaxseeds and walnuts.

The chapter finishes with the reminder that the journey of pregnancy nutrition extends beyond simply sustenance; it's a deliberate acceptance of nourishment that feeds both you and your baby. By navigating the nuances of unique dietary needs, recognizing food safety, and avoiding dangerous chemicals, you're participating in the establishment of a caring environment for new life.

CHAPTER NINE

Gestational Diabetes and Nutrition: Balancing Blood Sugar

In the delicate tapestry of pregnancy, the thread of gestational diabetes weaves its tale, calling for heightened awareness and a thoughtful diet. This section digs into the art of maintaining blood sugar levels through nutrition, including carbohydrate management and monitoring approaches.

- **Managing Blood Sugar Levels with Diet**

Gestational diabetes, a disorder that develops during pregnancy, demands a careful tango between food and blood sugar control. This chapter celebrates the art of constructing a diet that not only supports your body and your baby but also maintains consistent blood sugar levels.

Carbohydrates, the key macronutrient affecting blood sugar, play a vital role in gestational diabetes treatment. Balancing carbohydrate intake throughout meals and snacks can help reduce spikes and dips in blood sugar levels.

Embrace complex carbs, which release glucose gradually into your system, delivering prolonged energy. Whole grains, legumes, and veggies become the building blocks of your meals, establishing a foundation of nutrients that reduces blood sugar swings.

Incorporate lean proteins and healthy fats, since they slow down the absorption of carbs, further maintaining stable blood sugar levels. These nutrients add to the enjoyment and fullness of your meals, ensuring you feel content while keeping your blood sugar in check.

The chapter takes you on a culinary tour, exploring dishes and meal ideas tailored to respond to the special demands of gestational diabetes. From colorful salads with a protein twist to substantial soups that balance tastes and minerals, these dishes not only fuel your body but also enrich your meals with creativity and taste.

- **Carbohydrate Management and Monitoring**

The adventure continues with a thorough dive into carbohydrate management—a compass guiding your decisions and quantities. Carbohydrate counting becomes a wonderful tool, helping you to make educated decisions about the meals you consume.

Working together with a certified dietician, you'll learn to analyze the carbohydrate content of various meals and modify your intake appropriately. Portion management and distribution become crucial techniques, helping you to space out carbohydrate-rich items throughout the day.

Monitoring your blood sugar levels becomes a critical element of your routine. This practice gives insights into how your body responds to different diets and helps discover patterns that could require change. Regular blood sugar readings help you to make timely alterations to your diet and maintain stable levels.

As you navigate the area of gestational diabetes and nutrition, realize that this journey is not one you walk alone. Your healthcare physician, registered dietitian, and support network become key allies in developing a diet that promotes the health of both you and your baby.

By adopting the concepts of blood sugar regulation via nutrition, you're engaged in an act of self-care that reverberates through the delicate journey of pregnancy. This chapter urges you to explore the balance between feeding and blood sugar regulation, constructing a route that honors both your well-being and the well-being of your kid.

CHAPTER TEN

Prenatal Supplements: Nourishing Beyond the Plate

Amidst the canvas of pregnancy nutrition, the palette of prenatal vitamins contributes crucial colors to the masterpiece of maternal health. This section unravels the significance of prenatal vitamins, analyzes their function in pregnancy, and walks you through the process of discussing supplements with your healthcare practitioner.

• The Role of Prenatal Vitamins

Prenatal vitamins emerge as a cornerstone in the field of prenatal nutrition. They are intended to bridge any gaps in nutrition, ensuring both you and your growing baby receive the required vitamins and minerals for healthy growth.

While a balanced diet provides the foundation of your nutritional journey, the demands of pregnancy can occasionally lead to higher requirements for particular nutrients. Prenatal vitamins operate as a safety net, providing a dependable dose of vital nutrients such as folic acid, iron, calcium, and vitamin D.

Folic acid, for instance, plays a crucial function in avoiding neural tube abnormalities in the developing baby. Iron promotes the synthesis of red blood cells, fighting the danger of anemia. Calcium helps to strengthen bones and teeth, while vitamin D aids in their absorption.

The chapter looks into each of these critical nutrients, giving insights into their roles and the ramifications of their deficits during pregnancy. By knowing their significance, you're enabled to treat prenatal vitamins as a valuable ally in your journey.

• Discussing Supplements with Your Healthcare Provider

The trip into the domain of prenatal vitamins begins with a conversation—a discourse between you and your healthcare practitioner. This chapter leads you through the process of considering supplements, enabling you to make educated selections that match your unique needs.

Initiate the conversation with your healthcare professional early in your pregnancy experience. Their counsel can help you pick a prenatal vitamin that matches your requirements. Factors such as your nutrition, medical history, and any pre-existing diseases are evaluated in this decision-making process.

The chapter includes a list of questions to consider when discussing supplements with your healthcare professional. From inquiries about the optimal dose to potential interactions with other drugs, these questions equip you to engage in a detailed and meaningful dialogue.

Remember that your healthcare practitioner is your partner in your journey, delivering insights that are suited to your circumstances. Their experience ensures that the supplements you purchase complement your dietary choices and give the assistance your body needs throughout pregnancy.

As you explore into the realm of prenatal vitamins, know that they play a harmonic function alongside your dietary choices. They operate like a symphony conductor, overseeing the orchestration of nutrients that nourish both you and your kid.

By knowing the function of prenatal vitamins and tackling the issue of supplements alongside your healthcare professional, you're embracing a complete approach to pregnancy nourishment. This chapter asks you to establish a relationship with both your body and your healthcare provider, constructing a symphony of health that echoes throughout the journey of pregnancy.

CHAPTER ELEVEN

Healthy Weight Gain and Exercise: Nurturing Your Body's Balance

In the choreography of pregnancy, the steps of healthy weight gain and mindful exercise blend to produce a dance that celebrates the well-being of both you and your baby. This part discusses the art of reaching healthy weight gain objectives and leads you through safe and effective pregnant activities.

- **Achieving Healthy Weight Gain Goals**

Pregnancy signifies a moment of amazing transformation—a journey when your body fosters and maintains new life. The notion of healthy weight growth becomes an important aspect of this journey, reflecting not just your body's demands but also the well-being of your kid.

Healthy weight gain during pregnancy is a balance that differs from woman to woman. It's not just about the numbers on the scale, but about ensuring that you're supplying your body with the necessary nutrients to support the growth and development of your kid.

This chapter goes into the art of reaching healthy weight gain goals through mindful decisions. Embracing nutrient-dense meals, staying hydrated, and integrating a range of vitamins and minerals become crucial measures in this goal.

The road to healthy weight growth extends beyond the world of food; it also entails recognizing the messages your body sends. Paying attention to hunger cues and modifying your portion sizes accordingly helps you recognize your body's requirements without overindulging.

Furthermore, the chapter covers the psychological side of healthy weight growth, diving into the feelings that could develop throughout this transforming phase. Navigating body image and self-esteem becomes a vital aspect of accepting healthy weight gain with compassion and understanding.

- **Safe and Effective Prenatal Exercises**

The chapter switches to the world of movement—a vital part of pregnant well-being. Prenatal activities provide a symphony of advantages, from increasing your mood to enhancing flexibility and strength. Engaging in safe and effective activities throughout pregnancy can help to a smoother journey and an easier recovery postpartum.

Low-impact workouts including walking, swimming, and prenatal yoga become gentle companions in sustaining your physical well-being. They increase circulation, reduce pain, and support your body's fluctuating demands.

Strength exercise takes on a caring function during pregnancy, boosting muscle tone and maintaining your body's structure. Modified workouts that focus on stability and posture help to a stronger foundation.

Pelvic floor exercises, frequently disregarded yet vital, have a role in avoiding disorders such as incontinence and pelvic discomfort. These workouts strengthen the muscles that support your bladder, uterus, and bowels—essential during and after pregnancy.

The chapter finishes with the reminder that healthy weight growth and exercise interact to produce a symphony of well-being. By making conscious choices and implementing safe workouts, you're nourishing not just your body but also your relationship with your growing baby.

CHAPTER TWELVE

Postpartum Nutrition: Nurturing the Journey Beyond Birth

As the curtains rise on the postpartum phase, the focus moves to a new chapter of your journey—one that continues the symphony of nourishment and well-being. This section digs into the topic of postpartum nutrition, addressing your nutritional needs after birth and throughout nursing. It also takes you through the skill of gradually switching to a balanced diet.

• Nutritional Needs After Delivery and During Breastfeeding

The postpartum period is a time of regeneration and transition, defined by changes in your body and the obligations of caring for your infant. Nurturing your body with the correct nutrition during this time becomes crucial, supporting your recuperation and your baby's growth.

This chapter navigates through the special dietary demands you have after birth and while nursing. Nutrient-dense meals that offer energy and promote healing take center stage. Iron-rich meals help restore reserves lost during delivery, while protein helps tissue healing and immunological function.

Breastfeeding, a symphony of sustenance and connection, exerts additional demands on your body. The act of supplying nutrition to your infant involves an increased intake of calories, water, and certain nutrients. Calcium, vitamin D, and omega-3 fatty acids continue to play essential roles in maintaining your well-being and that of your kid.

The chapter takes you on a tour through the numerous nutrients your body demands postpartum. From the important role of protein in tissue regeneration to the necessity of iron in refilling your energy levels, you'll learn insights into how to fuel your body successfully throughout this time.

• Gradually Transitioning to a Balanced Diet

As you transition into the postpartum phase, the path of nurturing continues this time with a focus on both yourself and your infant. The shift to a balanced diet takes center stage, reflecting your changing demands and the developing nutritional requirements of your infant.

The chapter leads you through the art of gentle transition—a process that supports your body's recuperation while embracing your baby's developing demands. It's a delicate dance that balances the nutrients you supply via nursing with the energy you need for healing and caring for your kid.

Whole grains, lean meats, vibrant veggies, and healthy fats compose the palette of your postpartum diet. As you traverse the art of meal planning, consider meals that deliver prolonged energy, strengthen your immune system, and increase your mood.

Hydration, a loyal ally, is a vital feature of postpartum nutrition. Adequate fluid intake promotes breastfeeding and helps your body recover from the rigors of delivery. Herbal teas, water-rich fruits, and infused water become delicious methods to remain hydrated.

Conclusion:

The chapter finishes with a reminder that the journey of pregnancy nutrition extends into the world of postpartum when sustenance develops but continues to harmonize with your body's changing demands. By adopting the ideas of postpartum nutrition and gradually shifting to a balanced diet, you're building a tapestry of well-being that echoes through both your journey and that of your kid.

CHAPTER THIRTEEN

Recipes and Meal Ideas: Culinary Nourishment for Pregnancy

Embark on a gastronomic adventure that mixes sustenance and enjoyment in this chapter dedicated to dishes and meal ideas. From nutrient-rich meals that nourish your pregnancy to imaginative snacks that fulfill cravings, this area embraces the art of culinary creation for both you and your developing baby.

- ### Nutrient-Rich Meal Recipes for Pregnancy

The core of this chapter resides in the world of nutrient-rich meals that constitute the foundation of your pregnancy nutrition. These recipes are carefully created to supply the vitamins, minerals, and nutrition your body needs to support the remarkable adventure of creating a new life.

1. Hearty Breakfast Options

Berry Bliss Smoothie Bowl

Greet the morning with a blast of vigor in the shape of a Berry Bliss Smoothie Bowl. Blend mixed berries, a banana, Greek yogurt, and a splash of almond milk till smooth. Pour into a bowl and top with sliced almonds, chia seeds, and a drizzle of honey. This antioxidant-packed pleasure kick starts your day with energy and taste.

Energizing Oatmeal with Nuts and Seeds

For a pleasant morning, try a bowl of energetic oatmeal enhanced with nuts and seeds. Cook steel-cut oats with almond milk and a dash of cinnamon until creamy. Top with a mix of chopped nuts, pumpkin seeds, and a sprinkling of crushed flaxseed. This nutrient-dense meal fills your morning with fiber and healthy fats.

2. Wholesome Lunch Creations

Mediterranean Chickpea Salad

Lunchtime becomes a festival of flavors with a Mediterranean Chickpea Salad. Combine chickpeas, cherry tomatoes, cucumber, red onion, and Kalamata olives. Drizzle with olive oil, lemon juice, and a pinch of oregano. Finish with crumbled feta cheese for a flavor of the Mediterranean that's loaded with protein and colorful greens.

Grilled Vegetable Quinoa Bowl

Craft a hearty lunch with a Grilled Vegetable Quinoa Bowl. Grill a variety of vibrant veggies, from bell peppers to zucchini, then place them above a bed of cooked quinoa. Drizzle with balsamic vinaigrette and sprinkle with fresh herbs. This nutrient-packed dish delivers a delicious combination of tastes and textures.

● Snack Ideas to Satisfy Cravings

Indulge your pregnant cravings with a range of healthful and enjoyable foods meant to curb your demands while healing your body.

1. Crunchy Delights

Roasted Chickpeas with Spices

Roasted Chickpeas with Spices are a crispy and protein-packed snack that fulfills savory appetites. Toss cooked chickpeas with olive oil, cumin, paprika, and a touch of cayenne pepper. Roast till crispy for a wonderful snack that's rich in fiber and plant-based protein.

Trail Mix with a Twist

Create your own Trail Mix with a Twist by mixing nuts, seeds, and dried fruits. Add a sprinkling of dark chocolate chips for a bit of sweetness. This personalized snack includes a combination of healthy fats, antioxidants, and energy-boosting elements.

2. Sweet Gratification

Apple Slices with Nut Butter

For a delicious and fulfilling treat, enjoy Apple Slices with Nut Butter. Slice crisp apple slices and combine them with almond or peanut butter. The mix of fiber and healthy fats keeps you nourished and energized.

Greek Yogurt Parfait

Craft a Greek Yogurt Parfait by stacking Greek yogurt with fresh berries and a sprinkling of oats. This wonderful mix delivers a balance of protein, vitamins, and a touch of sweetness.

From stimulating breakfasts to comforting lunches, these dishes reflect the various tastes and nutritional demands of pregnancy. They weave tastes and minerals into a symphony of nutrition that follows you on this magnificent voyage.

CHAPTER FOURTEEN

Frequently Asked Questions: Navigating Common Nutrition Concerns

In the world of pregnancy nutrition, questions often emerge, and this chapter is dedicated to resolving those doubts that remain in the minds of pregnant women. From common nutrition concerns to professional solutions that give clarity, this area acts as a guiding light, helping you to make educated decisions for both your well-being and the health of your kid.

• Addressing Common Nutrition Concerns

This section provides a compass that helps you through the maze of typical dietary difficulties during pregnancy. Here, we examine the questions that resound in the minds of many mothers-to-be, giving insights and counsel to reduce fears and doubts.

1. Can I Continue to Enjoy Coffee?

One of the most popular inquiries is to drink coffee during pregnancy. We dig into the realm of coffee, dissecting the science behind its impact on you and your kid. We discuss the appropriate limits for caffeine use and provide advice for thoughtful consumption that corresponds with your well-being and the requirements of your growing kid.

The chapter discusses the issues of caffeine's influence on pregnancy, emphasizing the urge for that morning cup of comfort while underlining the necessity for moderation. Our purpose is to allow you to taste your favorite coffee in a way that respects your body's shifting dynamics.

2. Dealing with Digestive Discomfort

Pregnancy typically brings about adjustments in digestion that can cause pain. From heartburn to bloating and constipation, these changes might be baffling. In this area, we give solutions to address these typical discomforts, ranging from dietary modifications to lifestyle activities that improve digestive ease.

The investigation of digestive pain is a complete trip that touches on the need for water, mindful eating, and moderate movement. By giving insights into these problems, we want to lead you through the maze of pregnancy-related digestive changes with a sense of empowerment and pragmatism.

3. Cravings vs. Nutritional Needs

Cravings are characteristic of pregnancy, but decoding their message may be a mystery. In this section, we dig into the complex relationship between desires and nutritional demands. By investigating the science behind these desires, we give a different viewpoint on how your body communicates its necessities.

The chapter looks into the science of cravings, highlighting how your body's shifting nutritional demands could emerge as unique urges. Through this understanding, we enable you to negotiate cravings with awareness and make choices that suit both your body's requirements and your taste preferences.

• Expert Answers to Reader Questions

This area is a treasured resource of professional views, delivering solutions to the issues that readers like you have submitted. We've leaned into the experience of dietitians, obstetricians, and specialists to give authoritative solutions that light your path toward educated decisions.

1. Is it Safe to Consume Seafood During Pregnancy?

The ocean's wealth brings both nutrition and danger for expecting moms. In this part, we approach the seafood conundrum with clarity. We shed light on the forms of seafood that deliver critical nutrients while limiting potential dangers. Through professional insights, you'll uncover a plan for enjoying seafood that corresponds with the health of both you and your kid.

This investigation of seafood eating during pregnancy goes into the advantages of omega-3 fatty acids, the possible issues of mercury exposure, and actionable advice for selecting seafood that maximizes nutrition while decreasing risk.

2. How Can I Manage Weight Gain During Pregnancy?

Weight gain is a natural component of pregnancy, but its management demands a balanced approach. This part relies upon professional viewpoints to give insights regarding healthy weight gain objectives, techniques for maintaining a wholesome diet, and the necessity of embracing your body's changes.

Navigating the issue of weight increase during pregnancy demands compassion and accurate information. By giving professional viewpoints and practical guidance, we offer a comprehensive approach to controlling weight gain in a way that improves both your health and the well-being of your growing kid.

3. Unraveling the Mysteries of Food Aversions

Food aversions may be puzzling, affecting taste preferences and cooking practices. In this area, our experts give help in identifying and managing these fluctuations in taste preferences. Discover strategies to handle aversions while ensuring your nutritional needs are satisfied.

The investigation of food aversions is a caring path that respects the intricate interplay between hormones and taste during pregnancy. By giving techniques to work past aversions while still acquiring necessary nutrients, we enable you to accept the intricacies of your developing palette.

From drinking coffee to managing addictions, these questions and professional responses build a bridge between curiosity and clarity. They help you to sail the oceans of pregnancy nutrition with confidence, enhancing your experience with knowledge and insight.

Conclusion:

Nourishing the Journey of Pregnancy

The journey of pregnancy is a unique passage filled with expectation, transformation and a strong connection to the birth of new life. Throughout this book, "Real Food for Pregnancy," we've embarked on a trip together, delving into the area of nutrition as a cornerstone of this wonderful adventure. As we draw this trip to a conclusion, let us reflect on the lessons learned, insights acquired, and the nurturing route that lies ahead.

From the very first pages, we set out to study the tremendous influence of diet on the extraordinary journey of pregnancy. With each passing chapter, we've stitched together a tapestry of knowledge, offering evidence-based information that empowers pregnant moms to make educated decisions for their well-being and the well-being of their growing kids.

We've traveled through the fundamentals of constructing a balanced diet, recognizing the relevance of important nutrients, and handling the issues that may occur, from cravings and food aversions to gestational diabetes. In each inquiry, we've been guided by the concept of embracing "real food," realizing that the cornerstone of sustenance rests in entire, nutrient-dense ingredients that maintain both body and spirit.

Our research brought us to the heart of the kitchen, where nutrient-rich meal recipes were formed, and snack ideas evolved to fulfill appetites with knowledge and purpose. Through the pages of this book, we've learned that food isn't only about fuelling the body, but also about nurturing the soul, enjoying tastes, and relishing each mouthful as a link to the beautiful adventure of pregnancy.

Frequently asked questions lighted our route, answering common concerns with professional insights that spanned gaps of ambiguity. We walked through complexity, whether it was the balance of coffee intake, the skill of managing weight gain or comprehending the nuanced dance between appetites and nutritional demands.

Through the range of these debates, one unifying issue emerged: the significance of empowerment. Empowerment to make decisions that accord with individual needs, preferences, and unique situations. Empowerment is to accept the changes that pregnancy brings and to handle them with grace and understanding. Empowerment to approach nourishment with awareness, intention, and the realization that nourishing oneself also supports the growing life inside.

As we complete this trip through "Real Food for Pregnancy," let us take on the wisdom learned, the knowledge given, and the embracing of "real food" as a loving companion. The adventure of pregnancy is not only nine months; it is a continual journey of transformation, development, and love.

May this book serve as a guidepost, a friend, and a source of empowerment as you continue down the road of pregnancy. May your decisions be enlightened by the information obtained inside these pages, and may your nutrition be a monument to the magnificent trip you are undertaking—one filled with optimism, wonder, and the power of sustaining both body and spirit.

As you move on, know that you are not alone. Your journey is backed by the wisdom of generations, the advice of specialists, and the love that surrounds you. You contain within you the power to nourish, nurture, and create. This journey is your own, and as you continue to make decisions built-in knowledge, and love, may it be a monument to the beauty of life's most incredible trip: the adventure of pregnancy.

In closing, let the pages of this book be a reminder that every mouthful you eat, every choice you make, is a step ahead on the path to sustaining your journey and enjoying the endless beauty of pregnancy.

With warmth and best wishes,
[Irina Fomina]